FROM MANAGING TO CONQUERING BLOOD DISORDERS

Expert Guide To Understanding Causes, Symptoms, And Modern Treatment Approaches For Optimal Health

DR. DASHIELL DANIEL

Disclaimer

This book, is intended to provide information and guidance on the subject matter and is not a substitute for professional medical advice, diagnosis, or treatment.

The author, is not a medical professional, and the content presented here is based on research, general knowledge, and expert guidance available at the time of writing.

The information in this book is provided with the understanding that the author and the publisher are not engaged in rendering medical, legal, or other professional services.

Any reliance on the information contained in this book is at the reader's own risk.

While every effort has been made to ensure the accuracy and completeness of the information presented, medical knowledge is constantly evolving, and new research may supersede the content in this book. The author and the publisher make no representations or warranties of any kind, express or implied, about the completeness, accuracy, reliability, suitability, or availability concerning the information, products, services, or related graphics contained in this book.

This book may contain references or mentions of individuals, products, websites, organizations, or other names for informational purposes only.

The author does not own or endorse any such entities mentioned in the book. Any resemblance to actual persons, living or dead, or actual events is purely coincidental.

Readers are encouraged to consult with qualified healthcare professionals for medical advice, diagnosis, and treatment tailored to their specific circumstances.

The author and the publisher disclaim any liability for any loss or risk, personal or otherwise, arising directly or indirectly from the use of the information presented in this book.

By reading this book, the reader acknowledges and agrees to the terms of this disclaimer.

Blood Disorders: Unveiling the Essence of Hematologic Health is a thorough manual that delves into the complexities of blood-related illnesses and clarifies the mysteries surrounding the life-giving substance that flows through our veins. This book's goal is not just to list problems; rather, it aims to provide readers with a thorough grasp of blood disorders. It is written for a wide range of readers, including medical experts and those who are just inquisitive about the intricacies of hematologic health.

The objective of the Book:

Blood Disorders' main goal is to provide researchers, students, and healthcare professionals with an invaluable resource by demystifying the world of hematopoietic disorders. Through an in-depth examination of the components, uses, and dysfunctions of blood, the book seeks to equip readers with the knowledge necessary for diagnosis, treatment, and the development of a nuanced understanding of the effects of blood disorders on people as well as communities.

The intended audience

This book is designed to satisfy the requirements of researchers, doctors, hematologists, and medical students who want to gain a thorough understanding of blood disorders.

Because of its accessibility, both experts and laypeople can profit from its ideas, making it a useful and adaptable resource in a variety of educational and medical contexts.

Synopsis of Blood Disorders:

The book begins with an overview of blood, breaking out its many parts and purposes.

Each chapter adds to a comprehensive understanding of hematologic health, covering everything from the fundamentals of blood disorders to a thorough examination of red and white blood cell abnormalities, platelet disorders, bleeding and clotting disorders, and uncommon blood problems.

The reader's comprehension is further enhanced by the inclusion of chapters on diagnosis, treatment, and living with a blood condition.

All things considered, Blood Disorders is a knowledge-bearing resource that illuminates the complex web of hematologic abnormalities and gives readers the skills they need to meet the problems these disorders present. The book ends with a forward-looking chapter on future trends and research, providing a glimpse into the current achievements and prospective prospects in the field of hematology and serving as a testament to the continual growth of medical knowledge.

First Of All

Blood disorders are a broad field of study that explores the complexities of hematological illnesses influencing the structure, function, and synthesis of blood components.

The medical specialty of haematology, which studies blood-related illnesses, includes a wide range of conditions, from benign to potentially fatal. The goal of this thorough investigation is to clarify the intricate pathophysiological mechanisms that underlie these illnesses, promoting a better comprehension of diagnosis, treatment options, and future research directions.

The Objective Of The Book

This book's main objective is to provide a thorough resource for haematology students, researchers, and healthcare professionals. The book attempts to give a comprehensive foundation for comprehending the origin, clinical symptoms, and therapeutic options connected with these problems by compiling a plethora of knowledge on numerous blood disorders. Additionally, the book aims to close the knowledge gap between fundamental science and clinical practice by providing insights that support evidence-based choices for the diagnosis and management of blood disorders.

The Intended Audience

A wide range of readers, including hematologists, oncologists, pathologists, medical students, and researchers with an interest in hematology, are intended to benefit from this book.

It is meant to be understandable to both novices and experts alike who are just starting in the complicated field of blood diseases. Through a straightforward and well-structured presentation of material, the book hopes to promote learning and be a useful resource for readers with varying degrees of experience in the subject.

Synopsis Of Blood Disorders

diseases affecting red blood cells (erythrocytes), white blood cells (leukocytes), platelets (thrombocytes), and the components of plasma are all included in the broad field of blood diseases. Anemias and hemoglobinopathies are examples of erythrocyte disorders that cause changes in red blood cell count, size, or function, which impede oxygen transfer. White blood cell disorders include leukemias, lymphomas, and myelomas.

These conditions are frequently characterized by unchecked proliferation and compromised immunological function. Conditions involving platelets and the clotting cascade include thrombocytopenia, thrombocythemia, and coagulation disorders.

Hematological malignancies comprise a substantial category of blood illnesses with a variety of subcategories, such as lymphoma and leukemia. These neoplastic disorders cause aberrant blood cell survival and proliferation as a result of genetic abnormalities and cellular process dysregulation.

Because of improvements in molecular and genetic research, the classification of these cancers is always changing and helps to clarify their pathophysiology.

Non-neoplastic blood diseases include a broad range of ailments in addition to cancers. Hemoglobinopathies, which include thalassemia and sickle cell disease, are characterized by structural variations in hemoglobin that compromise hemolysis and oxygen transport.

The immune system attacking blood cells causes autoimmune illnesses such as autoimmune hemolytic anemia (AIHA) and immune thrombocytopenic purpura (ITP).

Haemostasis is further complicated by inherited illnesses like hemophilia and von Willebrand disease, which impair normal blood clotting processes.

Blood diseases are diagnosed using a multidisciplinary approach that includes molecular analysis, imaging studies, laboratory testing, and clinical examination.

Complete blood counts, peripheral blood smears, coagulation profiles, and bone marrow exams are examples of hematological investigations.

Technological developments like genetic testing and flow cytometry have improved our capacity to identify blood problems at the molecular level, leading to more accurate diagnosis and focused treatment plans.

Blood problems can be treated in a variety of ways, depending on the underlying pathophysiology, severity, and nature of the ailment. Hematopoietic stem cell transplantation, pharmaceuticals, transfusions, and supportive care techniques are examples of therapeutic approaches.

The discipline is dynamic, and constant attempts are being made in research to find new therapeutic targets and improve treatment strategies.

To sum up, this book provides an extensive overview of the complex field of blood diseases.

It provides a comprehensive view of the difficulties and developments in the field of hematology by covering the various facets of erythrocyte, leukocyte, and platelet problems as well as hematological malignancies and non-neoplastic illnesses.

The book aims to provide a comprehensive understanding of blood disorders, which can be useful for healthcare professionals or students.

It also lays the foundation for future research endeavors and improved patient care.

CHAPTER ONE
UNDERSTANDING BLOOD AND ITS COMPONENTS

The complex and essential fluid known as blood is essential to the preservation of homeostasis in the human body. Blood flows via an extensive network of blood vessels, making up around 8% of the body weight, carrying nutrients and oxygen while expelling waste. It acts as a dynamic transport system to guarantee that different tissues and organs work as they should. Blood is made up of various cellular and non-cellular elements, each of which has a unique purpose and affects an individual's general health and well-being.

Blood's Composition

Blood's makeup is incredibly varied, consisting of both cellular and non-cellular components. Red blood cells (erythrocytes), white blood cells (leukocytes), and platelets (thrombocytes) are the constituents of a cell. Blood plasma is the straw-coloured liquid in which these cells are floating. White blood cells are critical for immunological protection, red blood cells provide oxygen, and platelets are necessary for blood coagulation. Blood plasma's non-cellular constituents include waste products, proteins, electrolytes, water, and hormones. The delicate equilibrium among these constituents is crucial for the appropriate operation of the cardiovascular system.

Blood Cell Functions

Red Blood Cells (RBCs): Also known as erythrocytes, red blood cells are the most prevalent biological component of blood and are mostly in charge of carrying oxygen. RBCs are filled with the iron-containing protein hemoglobin, which binds to oxygen in the lungs and releases it into the body's tissues. These cells' distinctive biconcave form increases the surface area available for oxygen exchange. Red blood cell disorders including sickle cell disease and anemia can have a major impact on oxygen transport, which can result in weakness, exhaustion, and other consequences.

White Blood Cells (WBCs): Often known as leukocytes, white blood cells are essential to the immune system because they protect the body from infections and external threats. White blood cells come in various varieties, each with a distinct purpose. Monocytes are involved in clearing away cellular debris, lymphocytes coordinate immune responses, and neutrophils are phagocytes that take up and break down microorganisms. White blood cell disorders, including leukemia or leukopenia, can weaken the immune system and leave the body vulnerable to infections and other health issues.

Platelets

Small cell fragments called platelets, sometimes known as thrombocytes, are essential for hemostasis and blood coagulation. When a blood vessel is damaged, platelets attach themselves to the spot and release chemicals that set off a chain of events that eventually form a clot.

This procedure encourages tissue regeneration and stops excessive bleeding. Hemophilia and thrombocytopenia are two platelet-related disorders that can cause aberrant bleeding tendencies or trouble forming clots, which can prolong bleeding after accidents.

Blood Plasma

The liquid portion of blood, known as blood plasma, is used by the body to carry cells and dissolved materials. Approximately 55% of the entire blood volume is made up of waste materials, proteins, water, electrolytes, and hormones.

The plasma proteins fibrinogen, globulins, and albumin are important for blood clotting, immunological response, and osmotic pressure maintenance. Hormones carried in plasma control a variety of physiological functions, and the electrolyte balance within the plasma is critical for healthy cellular function. Blood plasma disorders, such as dysproteinemia or hypoalbuminemia, can have a broad, systemic impact on the general health and function of the organism.

To sum up, blood is a complex fluid that is both dynamic and intricate, consisting of both non-cellular and cellular components. Comprehending the roles played by red blood cells, white blood cells, platelets, and blood plasma is crucial to grasp the physiological mechanisms that underpin general health. A person may develop any number of blood illnesses as a result of imbalances in these components, each of which presents a different set of difficulties and effects on an individual's overall health.

CHAPTER TWO
FUNDAMENTALS OF BLOOD DISORDERS

A wide range of medical problems that impact the makeup, functionality, and synthesis of blood components in the human body are collectively referred to as blood disorders.

The blood is an essential bodily fluid that helps the immune system function, maintain homeostasis, and carry nutrients, oxygen, and waste products.

Blood-related problems fall into three primary categories: clotting disorders, bleeding disorders, and anemia. Reduced hemoglobin or red blood cell levels result in anemia, which lowers the body's ability to carry oxygen. Unusual platelets or clotting factors cause bleeding disorders, which lead to poor blood clotting and excessive bleeding. Contrarily, clotting abnormalities result in aberrant blood clot formation, which may lead to embolism or thrombosis.

Meaning And Categorization

Blood disorders, often known as hemopathies or hematologic disorders, are a broad category of illnesses that impact the blood and its constituent parts. Genetic mutations, acquired causes, or a combination of the two may be the cause of these illnesses. Hematologic illnesses can be broadly categorized as either malignant or benign. Anemias, clotting issues, and other non-cancerous blood cell-affecting illnesses are examples of benign disorders.

The majority of malignant illnesses are blood malignancies, including myeloma, lymphoma, and leukemia. Disorders affecting particular blood components, such as platelets, plasma proteins, white blood cells, and red blood cells, are also included in the classification. Comprehending the exact categorization is essential for precise diagnosis and the creation of focused therapeutic approaches.

Reasons And Danger Factors

Blood diseases have a variety of underlying medical issues, environmental variables, genetic predispositions, and other factors.

Genetic illnesses such as hemophilia, thalassemia, and sickle cell anemia can be caused by inherited genetic mutations. Toxin exposure, infections, autoimmune reactions, and dietary deficits are examples of acquired factors.

Environmental factors combined with genetics can cause some blood diseases. Furthermore, there are risk factors that raise the possibility of blood problems developing.

The risk can be increased by age, family history, exposure to radiation or chemicals, and certain medical treatments like chemotherapy. It is crucial to comprehend these underlying causes to effectively prevent and treat blood diseases.

Typical Symptoms

Blood diseases can have a wide range of symptoms, depending on the particular type and severity of the condition. Typical signs of anemia include weakness, exhaustion, breathing difficulties, and pale skin. Excessive bleeding from small wounds, persistent bleeding following surgery, or spontaneous bruising are all possible signs of bleeding disorders.

On the other hand, aberrant blood clot formation brought on by coagulation disorders can result in symptoms like stroke, pulmonary embolism, and deep vein thrombosis. Increased vulnerability to infections may arise from modifications in the quantity or functionality of white blood cells.

In cancerous blood diseases such as leukemia and lymphoma, swelling of the lymph nodes, inexplicable weight loss, and chronic exhaustion are typical symptoms. It is essential to identify these symptoms to have an early diagnosis and prompt treatment for blood diseases.

learning the fundamentals of blood disorders entails having a thorough awareness of their definition, categorization, causes, and typical symptoms. This information is the cornerstone for efficiently diagnosing, treating, and managing these illnesses, which are essential components of hematological medicine and have a substantial positive impact on healthcare as a whole.

CHAPTER THREE
RED BLOOD CELL DISORDERS

Red blood cell diseases are a wide range of illnesses that negatively impact red blood cells (RBCs) ability to function normally. RBCs are essential parts of the circulatory system that carry oxygen throughout the body. Anemia is a common disorder in this category that is defined as a reduction in the amount or quality of red blood cells. The word "anemia" is general and includes several subcategories, each with its etiology and set of clinical symptoms.

<u>Anemia</u>

Anemia is a haematological condition characterized by a decrease in the number of red blood cells in circulation or a drop in hemoglobin concentration in blood, which results in a reduced ability to carry oxygen. Anemia has a complex etiology, with causes ranging from genetic factors to chronic diseases and dietary inadequacies. Weakness, exhaustion, pale skin, and dyspnea are typical symptoms. A comprehensive clinical assessment, blood testing, and even a bone marrow examination are all part of the diagnosis process. Depending on the underlying cause, several treatment approaches may be used, such as blood transfusions, nutritional supplements, or drugs that increase the formation of red blood cells.

Anemia Deficiency In Iron

Anemia due to iron deficiency is by far the most common type of anemia in the world. Low blood iron levels, which are essential for the formation of hemoglobin, cause this illness. Its development is attributed to several factors, including inadequate nutritional intake, poor iron absorption, chronic blood loss, and increased iron requirement at specific life phases. Iron deficiency anemia is clinically characterized by hypochromic and microcytic red blood cells.

Iron supplements, dietary changes, and, if necessary, treating the underlying cause are all part of the treatment.

Acute Vitamin Deficiency

Low amounts of vital vitamins necessary for healthy erythropoiesis lead to vitamin deficiency anemias. Notable reasons include deficits in vitamin B12 and folate. These vitamins are essential for the development of red blood cells and the creation of DNA. Vitamin B12 insufficiency can be caused by malabsorption problems or a lack of intrinsic factors (pernicious anemia), whereas folate deficiency might be caused by inadequate food intake or malabsorption. Vitamin levels are measured through blood testing for diagnosis, and the underlying reason and supplements are addressed for treatment.

Anemias Hemolytic:

A collection of illnesses known as hemolytic anemias is distinguished by the early lysis of red blood cells.

Anemia and related symptoms can result from this rapid degradation, which can happen extravascularly or intravascularly. Hemolytic anemias can result from acquired causes like autoimmune reactions and certain infections, as well as inherited disorders like sickle cell disease and thalassemia. Treatment includes supportive care, blood transfusions in extreme situations, and management of underlying problems.

Sickle Cell Disease

A genetic hemoglobinopathy known as sickle cell disease is caused by aberrant hemoglobin S, which causes red blood cells to form stiff, crescent-shaped clots. Because of this changed morphology, normal blood flow is impeded, which can lead to vaso-occlusive episodes and pain crises.

Because heterozygous carriers have some protection against malaria, sickle cell disease is more common in populations where the disease is more prevalent. Pain alleviation, avoiding complications, and, in extreme situations, hematopoietic stem cell transplantation are the main goals of management.

Thalassemia

A class of hereditary illnesses known as thalassemia is defined by a deficiency in the synthesis of hemoglobin subunits, which results in an imbalance in the creation of the globin chain. Increased red blood cell death and inefficient erythropoiesis are the outcomes of this imbalance. The two kinds of thalassemia are alpha and beta, based on which globin chain is impacted.

Clinical signs might range from carriers who show no symptoms to severe anemias that need frequent blood transfusions. The main methods of treating thalassemia include genetic counseling, supportive care, and, in certain situations, bone marrow transplantation.

In conclusion, a broad range of illnesses that have a substantial influence on red blood cell function are collectively referred to as red blood cell disorders.

Key conditions in this area include anemia, iron-deficiency anemia, vitamin deficiency anemias, hemolytic anemias, sickle cell disease, and thalassemia, each of which has a unique etiology, clinical manifestation, and therapy approach. For proper diagnosis, treatment, and continuous research to enhance treatments, a thorough understanding of these illnesses is essential.

CHAPTER FOUR
DISORDERS OF WHITE BLOOD CELLS

White blood cell disorders are a broad category of illnesses that impact the generation, performance, and life expectancy of white blood cells (WBCs), which are essential constituents of the immune system. These illnesses can present as lymphomas or leukemias, each of which has unique subgroups and traits. Comprehending these ailments is essential for precise diagnosis, prognosis, and management.

Leukemia

A class of blood malignancies known as leukemia is distinguished by the uncontrollably high growth of immature white blood cells. The malignancy known as acute lymphoblastic leukemia (ALL) mostly attacks lymphoid cells and progresses quickly. It is common in kids and needs to be treated right away.

On the other hand, mature lymphocytes are the primary target of Chronic Lymphocytic Leukemia (CLL), a slowly developing leukemia that usually appears in elderly persons. Myeloid cells proliferate quickly in acute myeloid leukemia (AML), which can affect both adults and children. The hallmark of chronic myeloid leukemia (CML) is an excess of myeloid cells that build up in the blood and bone marrow as aberrant white blood cells.

The lymphoma

Cancers called lymphomas start in the lymphatic system, which includes the bone marrow, spleen, thymus, and lymph nodes. Named for Thomas Hodgkin, Hodgkin's lymphoma is a unique type of lymphoma that is defined by the presence of Reed-Sternberg cells. This subtype distinctively progresses via lymph nodes and is rather uncommon. The group of lymphomas known as non-Hodgkin's lymphoma (NHL) is more varied, with different subtypes displaying distinct clinical characteristics.

Different phases of lymphocyte development can be impacted by NHL, resulting in a variety of presentations and prognoses.

All, Or Acute Lymphoblastic Leukemia:

One of the hallmarks of ALL leukemia is the unchecked growth of immature lymphoblasts. Though it can strike adults as well, children are the main victims of this aggressive disease.

Because ALL frequently manifests quickly, immediate medical intervention is required. Anemia, thrombocytopenia, and a weakened immune system are the results of aberrant lymphoblasts pushing away healthy blood cells in the bone marrow, where it all begins.

Treatment strategies are heavily influenced by the genetic and molecular features of ALL, with targeted medicines becoming more and more critical to improving results.

Leukemia Chronic Lymphocytic (Cll)

B lymphocytes are the main target of CLL, a slowly developing leukemia that is more common in elderly persons. The illness frequently shows no symptoms, and it could be unintentionally found via normal blood tests. CLL cells build up in the blood and bone marrow, impairing immunological function and causing overpopulation. Although CLL is usually a slow-moving disease, in some situations it can progress more quickly and require medical attention. Chemotherapy, immunotherapy, watchful waiting for asymptomatic patients, and targeted medicines that try to interfere with particular pathways involved in CLL cell survival are some of the treatment approaches for CLL.

Leukemia Acute Myeloid (Aml)

The unchecked growth of myeloid precursor cells in the bone marrow is a defining feature of acute myeloid leukemia (AML), a malignancy that advances quickly. Although it can happen at any age, older persons are more likely to experience it. Because normal blood cell synthesis is suppressed, the condition frequently manifests as exhaustion, bruises, and recurring infections. AML is divided into many subtypes according to the genetic abnormalities that are present and the particular cell lineage that is impacted. To achieve a long-term remission, treatment usually entails intense chemotherapy. In certain instances, stem cell transplantation may also be attempted.

Leukemia Chronic Myeloid (Cml)

One of the hallmarks of CML, a myeloproliferative disease, is the aberrant growth of myeloid cells in the bone marrow, especially granulocytes.

The Philadelphia chromosome, which results from a translocation between chromosomes 9 and 22, is the defining feature of CML. The BCR-ABL fusion gene, which promotes unchecked cell proliferation, is formed as a result of this translocation.

There are three stages to CML: blast crisis, accelerated, and chronic. Since the discovery of tyrosine kinase inhibitors (TKIs), which directly target the BCR-ABL protein and offer many patients efficient and well-tolerated therapy, CML treatment options have undergone a substantial evolution.

Hodgkin's Lymphoma

Reed-Sternberg cells, giant aberrant cells present in afflicted lymph nodes, are a distinctive feature of Hodgkin's lymphoma. Typically, this uncommon lymphoma manifests as weight loss, nocturnal sweats, and painless lymph node swelling. There are two primary kinds of Hodgkin's lymphoma: nodular lymphocyte-predominant Hodgkin lymphoma (NLPHL) and classical Hodgkin lymphoma (cHL). Depending on the stage and subtype of the disease, treatment options for Hodgkin's lymphoma may include immunotherapy, chemotherapy, radiation therapy, and stem cell transplantation.

Different Types Of Lymphoma

A diverse collection of lymphoid cancers, non-Hodgkin's lymphoma (NHL) is not the same as Hodgkin's lymphoma since it does not contain Reed-Sternberg cells. Natural killer cells, B cells, or T cells can give rise to NHL, which can then split into a wide variety of subtypes with unique clinical characteristics. NHL has a complex etiology that includes immunologic, genetic, and environmental components. Histopathological examination is the primary diagnostic tool; treatment options are based on the subtype, stage, and unique patient characteristics. Chemotherapy, immunotherapy, radiation therapy, and, in certain situations, stem cell transplantation are examples of therapeutic techniques.

Finally, it should be noted that white blood cell diseases cover a wide range of illnesses, from aggressive and acute leukemias to lymphomas with a variety of clinical presentations.

Comprehending the unique characteristics of every condition is crucial for precise diagnosis and customization of suitable therapeutic approaches. Targeted medicines have revolutionized the management of many conditions and improved results for many patients because of advancements in molecular and genetic research. Our understanding of the fundamental causes of white blood cell diseases is still being deepened by ongoing research, which gives us hope for future advancements in both diagnosis and therapy.

CHAPTER FIVE
DISORDERS OF PLATES

A wide range of illnesses are referred to as platelet disorders because they impair the proper operation of platelets, which are essential components of blood that aid in clotting.

When blood vessels are damaged, platelets, often referred to as thrombocytes, are essential for maintaining hemostasis and limiting excessive bleeding. Von Willebrand disease, hemophilia, and thrombocytopenia are three serious platelet diseases.

Thrombocytopenia

A low quantity of platelets in the blood causes thrombocytopenia, a disorder that impairs blood clotting. Because platelets are essential for creating a plug at the site of blood vessel damage, bleeding tendencies tend to worsen when their count falls below normal ranges, which are normally less than 150,000 platelets per microliter of blood. Thrombocytopenia can have a variety of causes, such as immune system reactions, infections, medicines, bone marrow diseases, and genetic factors. A common type of thrombocytopenia called immune thrombocytopenia (ITP) occurs when the immune system unintentionally targets and kills platelets. Blood tests are used in diagnosis to measure platelet count and find underlying reasons. Treating the underlying reason, taking drugs to increase platelet production, or, in extreme situations, receiving platelet transfusions are among possible treatment options.

Blood Clotting

Factor VIII (Hemophilia A) or Factor IX (Hemophilia B) deficiencies or absences are the main clotting factors associated with hemophilia, a genetic bleeding condition. Proteins called coagulation factors are necessary for blood clotting; a lack of them causes prolonged bleeding episodes on the inside as well as the outside. Usually an X-linked recessive condition, hemophilia primarily affects men. After small injuries, patients may experience prolonged bleeding or spontaneous bleeding. Common side effects include bleeding from the joints and muscles, which can cause chronic pain and, if untreated, damage to the joints. Blood tests to detect clotting factor levels are part of the diagnosis process. Treatment options include preventive measures, gene therapy in certain situations, and infusions to replace the defective clotting factor.

Von Willebrand Disease

Hemophilia is not the same as Von Willebrand Disease (VWD), another genetic bleeding illness. Von Willebrand factor (VWF), a protein essential to platelet adhesion and clotting factor stabilization, is either lacking or malfunctioning. Based on the severity of the VWF deficit, three forms of VWD are identified. Following surgery or an injury, symptoms might vary from minor bruising and nosebleeds to more serious bleeding episodes. Blood tests are used in diagnosis to evaluate VWF function and levels. Treatment options include clot-stabilizing drugs, desmopressin (DDAVP) to induce the release of stored VWF, or in more severe situations, VWF replacement therapy. A multidisciplinary strategy is necessary for managing VWD, taking into account the nature and severity of the illness.

Finally, platelet diseases including Von Willebrand Disease, thrombocytopenia, and hemophilia have a major effect on the delicate balance of blood clotting mechanisms. Effective management and better patient outcomes depend on having a thorough understanding of each disorder's underlying causes, diagnostic techniques, and suitable treatment options.

CHAPTER SIX
BLEEDING DISORDER

A class of medical illnesses known as bleeding disorders is defined by abnormal bleeding, which can be excessive or spontaneous in response to an injury. These conditions frequently entail abnormalities or shortages in blood clotting process components, impairing the body's capacity to generate a stable blood clot and successfully stop bleeding. A disruption in the complex balance between procoagulant and anticoagulant elements within the coagulation cascade is a common underlying component in bleeding disorders.

A person's haemostatic system is greatly impacted by bleeding disorders such as hemophilia, von Willebrand disease, and platelet disorders.

Reasons For Prolonged Bleeding

An essential component of treating bleeding problems is comprehending the reasons behind heavy bleeding. Genetic factors are often important since people can inherit deficits or abnormalities in clotting factors or platelet function. For example, hemophilia is an X-linked genetic condition that causes coagulation factors VIII (hemophilia A) or IX (hemophilia B) to be deficient. Vitamin K insufficiency, liver illness, and some drugs that may interfere with the manufacture or function of clotting components are acquired causes of heavy bleeding. Furthermore, antibodies against clotting factors may develop as a result of autoimmune illnesses, increasing the risk of excessive bleeding.

Different Bleeding Disorder Types

The range of illnesses with different etiologies and clinical presentations that make up bleeding disorders is broad. As previously said, hemophilia is a well-known hereditary bleeding illness that is divided into hemophilia A and B according to the deficiency of clotting factors. Another common bleeding ailment called von Willebrand disease is caused by a lack or malfunction of the von Willebrand factor, which is essential for platelet adhesion and clotting factor VIII stabilization. Hemostasis is hampered by platelet illnesses including immune thrombocytopenic purpura (ITP) and Bernard-Soulier syndrome, which alter platelet production or function. Because every bleeding problem is different, diagnosis and treatment must be customized for each one.

Options For Treatment

Restoring the delicate equilibrium of the haemostatic system and addressing the particular underlying cause are the two main goals of managing bleeding disorders. The mainstay of hemophilia treatment is replacement therapy with clotting factor concentrates, which replenishes the defective factor necessary for healthy blood coagulation. Desmopressin and von Willebrand factor concentrates are used to improve clotting factor function in cases of von Willebrand disease. Medication to increase platelet production or, in extreme situations, platelet transfusions may be necessary for platelet abnormalities. Supportive interventions, such as the use of antifibrinolytic drugs to stop clots from breaking down and blood component transfusions to treat acute bleeding episodes, may be used in addition to this focused therapy. Furthermore, by targeting the genetic foundation of several bleeding problems, advances in gene therapy hold hope for long-term remedies.

In conclusion, because of their complex pathophysiology and wide range of etiologies, bleeding diseases provide several difficulties for both patients and medical professionals.

 For bleeding disorders to be effectively managed and the quality of life for those who are affected to be improved, a complete understanding of the causes, kinds, and available treatments is essential. The field of bleeding problem management is constantly evolving due to ongoing research and technology breakthroughs, which gives hope for more specialized and creative therapeutic approaches in the future.

CHAPTER SEVEN

DISORDERS OF CROSSING

Anomalies in the process of blood clotting define clotting disorders, also referred to as coagulation disorders. Procoagulant and anticoagulant factors must be carefully balanced in this complex system to maintain appropriate hemostasis. Any perturbation to this balance may result in unsuitable clotting or excessive bleeding, which may contribute to a range of clinical symptoms. Clotting diseases affect people of all ages and can be either inherited or acquired.

DVT, or deep vein thrombosis:

A clotting condition known as deep vein thrombosis (DVT) is typified by the development of blood clots, or thrombi, in the body's deep veins, usually in the legs. Virchow's triad—blood stasis, hypercoagulability, and vascular damage—plays a role in the etiology. Numerous risk factors, such as extended immobility, surgery, trauma, and genetic predisposition, are linked to DVT.

DVT has serious clinical ramifications because clots can become dislodged and migrate to the lungs, where they can cause pulmonary embolism (PE), a potentially fatal illness. Compression stockings, anticoagulant treatment, and, in specific situations, interventional procedures are all part of the management methods for deep vein thrombosis.

PE, Or Pulmonary Embolism

A serious symptom of clotting problems is pulmonary embolism (PE), in which blood clots that usually originate in the legs' deep veins (DVT) go to the pulmonary arteries and restrict blood flow to the lungs. PE can cause hemoptysis, dyspnea, and chest discomfort, among other symptoms that can cause serious morbidity and death. PE can range in severity from asymptomatic cases to potentially fatal circumstances. Imaging tests like ventilation-perfusion scans and computed tomography pulmonary angiography (CTPA) are examples of diagnostic modalities. Anticoagulation is used in management to stop the spread of the clot, and in more serious situations, thrombolysis or embolectomy is performed.

DIC stands for disseminated intravascular coagulation.

The complicated and possibly fatal clotting condition known as disseminated intravascular coagulation (DIC) is defined by the systemic activation of coagulation factors, which results in extensive microvascular thrombosis.

This hypercoagulable state frequently results from an underlying illness such as sepsis, trauma, or cancer. Inversely, because consumptive coagulopathy in DIC causes clotting factors and platelets to be depleted, it might lead to bleeding problems. From minor test abnormalities to fulminant multi-organ failure, the clinical presentation can vary. Assessing clinical and laboratory indicators, such as fibrinogen levels, prothrombin time, and platelet count, is part of the diagnosis process.

The treatment of DIC involves several different approaches, including managing the coagulopathy with supportive measures, blood product infusions, and sometimes anticoagulation, as well as addressing the underlying cause.

for doctors to give prompt and efficient therapies, they must have a thorough awareness of clotting diseases, such as disseminated intravascular coagulation, pulmonary embolism, and deep vein thrombosis. A thorough approach to diagnosis and treatment is necessary due to the delicate balance of the coagulation system, taking into account the underlying causes and related consequences of these illnesses.

CHAPTER EIGHT
RARE BLOOD DISORDERS

Anemia Aplastic:

One rare and serious blood condition known as aplastic anemia is characterized by a lack of red blood cell synthesis in the bone marrow. Pancytopenia is the result of the bone marrow's inability to produce enough red, white, and platelet blood cells in this disease. The underlying pathology usually consists of injury to the bone marrow's hematopoietic stem cells, which reduces their capacity to create mature blood cells. Although this illness is frequently diagnosed as idiopathic, it can also be brought on by exposure to toxins, certain environmental variables, or the aftermath of autoimmune diseases. The clinical manifestations of aplastic anemia include exhaustion, heightened vulnerability to infections, and an elevated risk of bleeding as a result of a decrease in the quantity of functioning red blood cells.

Hematopoietic stem cell transplantation, immunosuppressive medication, and supportive care are among the treatment options used to control the disorder's symptoms and complications.

Hemoglobinuria Paroxysmal Nocturnal (Pnh)

A rare acquired blood condition called Paroxysmal Nocturnal Hemoglobinuria (PNH) is typified by an aberrant red blood cell breakdown. The main cause of it is a somatic mutation in the PIG-A gene, which results in the faulty blood cells that complement-mediated hemolysis can cause. Hemolysis, which occurs more frequently at night and releases free hemoglobin into the bloodstream, causes hemoglobinuria and is a characteristic of PNH. PNH patients may also develop thrombosis as a result of complement activation. Anemia, exhaustion, stomach pain, and black urine are examples of clinical symptoms. Flow cytometry, which measures the lack of glycosylphosphatidylinositol (GPI)-anchored proteins on the surface of blood cells, is frequently used to confirm the diagnosis. Complement inhibitors like eculizumab have completely changed the way PNH is managed since they provide a focused therapy strategy that targets the underlying complement dysregulation.

MDS, Or Myelodysplastic Syndromes

The diverse set of hematologic illnesses known as myelodysplastic syndromes (MDS) is defined by inadequate hematopoiesis, which results in dysplastic and defective blood cells. MDS is mostly related to bone marrow and is caused by chromosomal abnormalities or genetic alterations in hematopoietic stem cells. This leads to the generation of aberrant and immature blood cells, which increases the chance of developing acute myeloid leukemia (AML) and causes cytopenias.

There is a wide range in the clinical presentation, from asymptomatic cytopenias to signs of bone marrow failure, including infections, bleeding, and exhaustion. Several variables, such as the extent of cytopenia, the proportion of blasts in the bone marrow, and cytogenetic anomalies, are taken into consideration when classifying MDS patients. There are many different MDS treatment choices, and they are based on variables including patient characteristics and risk classification. For qualified patients, these could involve immunosuppressive medication, growth factors, transplanting hematopoietic stem cells, and supportive care. As new treatment techniques and targeted medicines are investigated, the management of MDS is changing.

diagnosing and treating unusual blood illnesses such as myelodysplastic syndromes (MDS), paroxysmal nocturnal hemoglobinuria (PNH), and aplastic anemia pose particular difficulties. Comprehending the fundamental pathophysiology of these conditions is essential for formulating efficacious therapy approaches.

The mechanisms underlying these uncommon blood illnesses have been better-understood thanks to developments in molecular and genetic research, opening the door to more specialized and individualized treatment modalities. Furthermore, continuous clinical studies and teamwork among medical professionals aid in the advancement of our comprehension and treatment of these intricate illnesses. The chances for better outcomes and a higher standard of living for those who are impacted by uncommon blood illnesses remain bright as we continue to understand their complexities.

CHAPTER NINE
DIAGNOSIS OF BLOOD DISORDERS

Blood problem diagnosis is a multifaceted and intricate procedure that requires a thorough understanding of clinical symptoms, hematological parameters, and cutting-edge diagnostic methods. A broad spectrum of illnesses is included in the term "blood disorders," such as anemias, leukemias, clotting issues, and other hematologic cancers. Hematological tests are essential to the first evaluation, and one of the most important tests is the complete blood count (CBC). The complete blood count (CBC) gives vital information about the red, white, and platelet components of blood, enabling medical professionals to recognize anomalies such as anemia, leukocytosis, or thrombocytopenia.

The foundation of diagnosing blood disorders is the use of blood tests and diagnostic techniques. In addition to CBC, other tests like serum protein electrophoresis, coagulation investigations, and peripheral blood smears offer insightful information about the precise nature of the illness. Examining blood smears, for example, makes it possible to spot aberrant cell morphology, which is essential for differentiating between leukemias and anemias. Conversely, coagulation investigations help identify clotting diseases such as von Willebrand disease and hemophilia.

Furthermore, the diagnosis of blood disorders has been completely transformed by the development of sophisticated diagnostic technology. Genetic mutations linked to a range of blood illnesses can be found using molecular techniques including fluorescence in situ hybridization (FISH) and polymerase chain reaction (PCR). These methods aid in the identification of focused treatment strategies in addition to improving diagnosis accuracy. Characterizing particular cell populations is made possible by the incorporation of flow cytometry into hematological diagnostics, which aids in the diagnosis of diseases such as lymphomas.

a methodical strategy combining conventional blood tests with state-of-the-art diagnostic technology is required for the identification of blood disorders. Through the use of an integrated method, physicians can not only determine whether a blood problem is present but also describe its particular characteristics, which helps to direct further treatment efforts.

Tests On Blood And Diagnostic Techniques

The diagnostic process for blood disorders is mostly based on blood tests and diagnostic procedures, which offer vital information on the physiological and pathological features of hematological problems. The primary blood test known as a complete blood count (CBC) evaluates the red blood cells (RBCs), white blood cells (WBCs), and platelets that make up blood. Variations in these characteristics can point to a variety of blood diseases, including thrombocytopenia's, leukemias, and anemias.

Another crucial diagnostic technique is peripheral blood smears, which provide an in-depth analysis of blood cell shape. By identifying aberrant cell sizes, shapes, and inclusions, this microscopic study facilitates the distinction of different blood diseases. For instance, sickle cell anemia is identified by the presence of sickle-shaped red blood cells on a peripheral blood smear.

Coagulation investigations are essential for the diagnosis of blood clotting disorders. Blood clotting capacity is assessed by tests like prothrombin time (PT) and activated partial thromboplastin time (aPTT), which are crucial in the diagnosis of diseases like hemophilia and disseminated intravascular coagulation (DIC). D-dimer testing can also reveal the existence of aberrant blood clot formation.

Serum protein electrophoresis is used to quantify and separate various blood proteins, such as immunoglobulins. When diagnosing diseases like multiple myeloma, which is characterized by an aberrant proliferation of plasma cells that produce monoclonal immunoglobulins, this test is helpful.

Molecular methods that concentrate on genetic and molecular markers are part of the rapidly changing field of blood disease diagnostics.

The amplification and detection of particular DNA sequences is made possible by the polymerase chain reaction (PCR), which helps identify genetic alterations linked to diseases like hemophilia and thalassemia. Another molecular method that helps identify chromosomal abnormalities connected to hematological malignancies is fluorescence in situ hybridization or FISH.

a variety of methods are used in blood tests and diagnostic processes that offer vital information for the identification and treatment of blood problems. These diagnostic tools, which range from sophisticated molecular tests to more conventional approaches like CBC and peripheral blood smears, provide to provide a thorough picture of hematological diseases and help doctors make decisions about patient care.

Imaging Methodologies

Imaging methods are essential for the diagnosis and treatment of blood disorders because they provide a non-invasive way to see the hematopoietic system's functional and structural features. Even though cellular and molecular abnormalities are the main causes of blood diseases, imaging is crucial for determining organ involvement, spotting consequences, and directing treatment approaches.

Ultrasound is one of the most frequently used imaging modalities since it can image blood vessels and organs in real time. In particular, Doppler ultrasound makes it possible to evaluate blood flow, which helps with the identification of diseases including vasculitis and deep vein thrombosis (DVT). Additionally, splenomegaly or hepatomegaly, which are common symptoms of specific blood disorders, can be seen using abdominal ultrasonography.

The spleen, bone marrow, and lymph nodes can all be seen in great detail in cross-sectional images of the body provided by computed tomography (CT) scans. CT scans are useful in guiding the staging of leukemia and lymphomas by assessing the amount of organ involvement. CT angiography is also used to evaluate vascular architecture and identify anomalies like thrombosis or aneurysms.

To evaluate soft tissues and organs, magnetic resonance imaging, or MRI, is especially useful.

It helps with the diagnosis of diseases including myeloproliferative disorders and bone marrow disorders by providing comprehensive images of the bone marrow. Furthermore, diffusion-weighted imaging and other functional MRI methods help characterize lesions and direct therapy decisions.

Because nuclear medicine methods can identify metabolic activity in tissues, such as positron emission tomography (PET) scans, are used in this regard. PET scans are useful for the detection of regions with elevated metabolic activity, which helps with the diagnosis and follow-up of hematologic malignancies such as lymphomas.

In conclusion, imaging techniques provide a non-invasive way to evaluate organ involvement, identify problems, and direct treatment plans for blood disorders, which is a complement to existing diagnostic procedures. From nuclear medicine and MRI to ultrasound and CT scans, these modalities add to a thorough diagnostic approach, improving our understanding of hematological disorders and enabling individualized patient management.

Genetic Examination

The use of genetic testing has become essential for the diagnosis, evaluation of risk, and treatment of many blood illnesses. Finding genetic mutations helps with early diagnosis, prognosis, and the creation of focused treatment strategies by shedding light on the underlying molecular pathways of various ailments.

Genetic testing is essential for the diagnosis of hemoglobinopathies, including thalassemia and sickle cell anemia. The identification of certain globin gene mutations is made possible by molecular methods such as DNA sequencing and polymerase chain reaction (PCR), which help doctors confirm diagnoses and assess the severity of patients' illnesses.

Genetic testing is also done for inherited clotting diseases such as von Willebrand disease and hemophilia. Accurate diagnosis and classification of these illnesses are made possible by the identification of pathogenic mutations by analysis of specific clotting factor genes. This genetic data is essential for determining the likelihood of bleeding issues and for directing the most suitable course of action.

Genetic testing is very beneficial to the field of hematologic malignancies, especially in the precision medicine age.

Genetic abnormalities linked to leukemia, lymphoma, and myeloma can be identified using chromosomal analysis, fluorescence in situ hybridization (FISH), and next-generation sequencing (NGS) techniques.

In addition to helping identify certain hematologic malignancy subtypes, this molecular profile directs the choice of targeted medicines, resulting in more efficient and individualized treatment modalities.

Genetic testing also affects counseling and screening within families. When a hereditary component is suspected, as in some cases of lymphomas or leukemias, determining genetic predispositions might help guide preventive measures and educate family members about their risk.

genetic testing has completely changed how blood disorders are diagnosed and treated. Genetic testing offers a clearer understanding of the underlying molecular basis of various illnesses, including hemoglobinopathies, coagulation disorders, and hematopoietic malignancies.

This information represents a paradigm shift in the treatment of blood disorders in the era of genomic medicine. It not only helps with precise diagnosis and risk assessment, but it also creates opportunities for tailored therapeutic approaches.

CHAPTER TEN
CARE AND SUPERVISION

Blood diseases are a broad category of illnesses that impact the make-up, functionality, or generation of blood components.

Effective management and treatment of these illnesses require a thorough grasp of the techniques used. Four main topics are covered in this discussion: medications, blood transfusions, bone marrow transplants, and supportive care and lifestyle modifications.

Drugs

For those with blood diseases, pharmaceutical therapy is essential for symptom relief, averting complications, and enhancing the general quality of life. Different pharmaceutical classes may be used, depending on the particular disorder.

For example, erythropoiesis-stimulating drugs or iron supplements may be recommended to promote the synthesis of red blood cells in anemic patients. In contrast, anticoagulants are frequently used to treat or prevent irregular blood clotting in diseases such as atrial fibrillation and deep vein thrombosis. The specific drug selected will depend on several criteria, including the patient's general health, the severity of the disorder, and the underlying pathology. It is frequently important to closely monitor and modify medication regimens to maximize therapeutic benefits and minimize potential side effects.

Transfusions Of Blood

Blood transfusions are an essential therapeutic approach for managing a range of blood illnesses, especially those that are typified by deficits in particular blood components. Transfusions of red blood cells are frequently used to treat anemia because they quickly increase the body's ability to carry oxygen. People with conditions like thrombocytopenia that impair platelet function or production require platelet transfusions. Additionally, disorders involving abnormalities in clotting factors might warrant plasma transfusions. Thorough donor screening, blood typing, and cross-matching protocols are essential for the safety and effectiveness of blood transfusions to reduce the possibility of transfusion responses. The availability and safety of blood products have improved due to advancements in blood banking technology and storage techniques, which have also improved patient outcomes for patients with different blood disorders.

Transplantation Of Bone Marrow

An innovative treatment option for some severe and resistant blood diseases is bone marrow transplantation. During this process, damaged or inoperable bone marrow is replaced with healthy hematopoietic stem cells infused into the body. Bone marrow transplants are frequently indicated for leukemia, lymphoma, and specific genetic diseases affecting the formation of red blood cells. Bone marrow transplant outcomes depend on several variables, including donor compatibility, conditioning schedules, and post-transplant care. Allogeneic transplants, which use donor cells, have a high risk of graft-versus-host disease but also can cure a patient completely. To reduce these hazards, autologous transplants—which use the patient's cells—are used in specific circumstances. Hematopoietic stem cell transplantation is an ever-evolving area that is expanding the range of blood illnesses that can be treated while also improving technique.

Modifications To Lifestyle And Supportive Care

In addition to pharmaceutical treatments, supportive care, and lifestyle changes are essential components of blood condition management. Dietary changes could be advised, especially if anemia is caused by dietary deficits. Adopting healthier lifestyle habits, such as regular exercise, staying hydrated, and avoiding extended periods of immobility, may be beneficial for patients with clotting issues. In addition to providing physical care, supportive care measures also include psychosocial support, which attends to the emotional and mental health of those who are coping with chronic blood problems.

Support groups, counseling, and coping technique instruction all play a major role in improving patients' and their families' overall quality of life. Palliative care may occasionally be combined with other therapies to improve comfort and reduce symptoms for patients with severe or terminal blood diseases.

the management and treatment of blood diseases necessitate a multimodal strategy that includes modern medical treatments such as bone marrow transplants, pharmaceuticals, transfusion medicine, and comprehensive supportive care.

The ever-evolving field of medicine is opening up new treatment options, which gives those with various blood problems hope for better outcomes and a higher standard of living.

CHAPTER ELEVEN
LIVING WITH A BLOOD DISORDER

Blood condition sufferers deal with a special set of difficulties that have a big influence on their day-to-day life. Anemia, hemophilia, leukemia, and different clotting disorders are only a few of the illnesses that fall within the broad category of blood disorders. Living with a blood condition is a complicated and diverse experience.

Patients frequently face difficulties navigating the complexities of their condition on a social, emotional, and physical level. People with blood diseases need to learn resilience and adaptability to manage their symptoms, adhere to treatment plans, and deal with the uncertainty surrounding the course of their disease.

Depending on the exact ailment, blood disorders can have quite different physical effects. For example, anemia can cause weakness, exhaustion, and dyspnea, which can make it difficult for a person to carry out daily tasks. However, coagulation abnormalities may make people more vulnerable to heavy bleeding, which can have detrimental effects on their health. Living with these physical manifestations necessitates proactive treatment, such as routine check-ups with the doctor, taking prescribed drugs as directed, and making lifestyle changes to reduce the worsening of symptoms.

The psychological effects of a blood condition can be rather severe emotionally. Individuals may struggle with despair, anxiety, or dread of health-related consequences. Many blood problems are chronic, meaning that continuous emotional support and coping skills are required.

Creating a positive view and strengthening one's resilience become essential components of overcoming emotional obstacles. The effects on interpersonal relationships, such as those in families and social settings, further complicate the emotional experience of having a blood condition.

Socially, people with blood problems frequently have to navigate a world that may be unaware of or lacking in understanding. Feelings of stigmatization or isolation may result from the need for accommodations, such as time off work for medical appointments or modifications to physical activities. It becomes essential to educate the general public about blood disorders to promote inclusivity and understanding. People with blood disorders need social support, such as advocacy groups and community organizations, to feel understood and accepted.

Adaptive Techniques

Managing a blood issue necessitates a multimodal strategy that takes into account the social, emotional, and physical aspects of the illness.

The development of efficient self-management techniques is a crucial component of coping. Patients are frequently urged to understand their conditions, take an active role in decision-making, and become actively involved in their healthcare.

A sense of control over their care and health is fostered by this empowerment.

A key element of coping mechanisms for blood diseases is medical care. Taking prescribed drugs as directed, keeping an eye on blood parameters regularly, and seeking medical attention when needed are crucial for treating symptoms and averting consequences. To develop personalized treatment programs that take into account their unique requirements and circumstances, patients and their healthcare professionals must collaborate closely.

Living changes are essential for managing blood diseases, in addition to medical treatment. This could entail altering one's diet, starting an exercise program, and abstaining from certain activities that might make symptoms worse. For instance, to reduce the chance of bleeding after an injury, people with coagulation issues could be recommended to stay away from contact sports. These lifestyle changes are intended to improve general well-being and are customized to the specific needs of each patient.

Coping tactics need psychosocial support. Psychologists and counselors, among other mental health providers, can help people create coping strategies to manage the emotional difficulties that come with having a blood condition.

Support groups offer a forum for people to interact with others going through comparable situations, exchanging stories and coping mechanisms.

Peer support lessens feelings of loneliness and promotes a sense of community.

Initiatives for education are also an essential component of coping mechanisms. Patients are better able to make decisions and take an active role in their care when they are well informed about their disease, available treatments, and potential obstacles. Written and digital educational materials help people with blood diseases become more health-literate and help spread accurate information.

Support Teams:

Support groups offer a sense of community, reciprocal encouragement, and shared understanding, making them vital tools for those with blood diseases. These groups, whether they are online or in person, provide a forum for people to connect with others going through comparable struggles. Members of these groups can benefit greatly from the sharing of experiences, coping mechanisms, and emotional support with others who suffer from blood disorders.

Individuals looking for in-person encounters can find a concrete feeling of community in in-person support groups. These groups frequently get together regularly, giving members the chance to talk about treatment alternatives, exchange experiences, and get emotional support from one another. By normalizing the difficulties connected with blood disorders and fostering a sense of belonging, the communal element helps people feel less alone.

In the digital age, online support groups have grown in popularity as they offer a virtual platform for people to communicate with each other wherever in the world. Participants can participate in conversations and access resources from the comfort of their homes thanks to the flexibility provided by the online format.

These online forums serve a wide variety of blood illnesses, so those with uncommon conditions can still access pertinent information and support.

Support groups enable people with blood diseases to share helpful tips on coping with day-to-day issues. Frequently, participants offer their perspectives on managing the side effects of treatment, navigating healthcare systems, and addressing the emotional elements of their conditions. These organizations' pooled knowledge enables people to take an active role in self-management and empowers them to become advocates for their health.

Life Quality

For people with blood disorders, quality of life refers to a comprehensive evaluation of health that extends beyond symptom treatment. Despite the difficulties brought on by the blood condition, it takes into account all facets of a person's life— physical, emotional, social, and psychological—to maximize total contentment and satisfaction.

Physically speaking, strategies to improve quality of life could include minimizing adverse effects from treatment plans, successfully managing symptoms, and fostering general health and well-being. Care plans may include pain management techniques, assistive technology, and rehabilitation services to help people with blood problems operate better daily.

A vital element of quality of life is emotional health. The provision of mental health assistance, such as counseling and psychotherapy, is essential in managing the emotional difficulties arising from chronic illnesses. An enhanced emotional state generally is facilitated by coping skills, stress management tactics, and anxiety and depression management approaches.

Blood disorder patients' quality of life is greatly impacted by social circumstances. Peers, relatives, and other supportive social networks all help to foster a feeling of community and lessen feelings of loneliness. Engaging in social activities and attending community events helps improve social integration and mitigate the possibility of social disengagement that could arise from the difficulties of managing a blood condition.

Another aspect of quality of life is having access to jobs and educational possibilities. Because of their health, people with blood diseases may encounter particular difficulties in going to school or keeping a job. By encouraging independence and self-sufficiency, inclusive policies, employment adjustments, and educational support can have a positive effect on people's quality of life.

In the end, a patient-centered evaluation of the quality of life for people with blood diseases should take into account the goals, values, and preferences of the individual. To customize interventions to match the patient's priorities, shared decision-making between patients and healthcare providers is essential. To maximize the quality of life for people with blood diseases, a thorough, multidisciplinary approach that takes into account their physical, emotional, social, and psychological needs is necessary.

CHAPTER TWELVE
RESEARCH AND FUTURE TRENDS

Blood disease research is expected to be dynamic and revolutionary in the future, with a focus on a few critical areas that have the potential to significantly advance our knowledge of and ability to treat these conditions. The growing focus on customized medicine, which adjusts therapies based on each patient's particular genetic composition and illness features, is one notable trend. The identification of particular genetic markers linked to a range of blood illnesses is being made possible by genomic studies, which will allow for targeted medicines with higher efficacy and fewer adverse effects. We will be able to forecast illness development and treatment outcomes even more precisely as long as artificial intelligence and machine learning are integrated into the analysis of large datasets, as technology advances.

The investigation of immunotherapy strategies is a remarkable development in the field of blood disorders research. By using the immune system's ability to identify and destroy cancerous cells, immunotherapeutic treatments—like CAR-T cell therapy—have shown impressive results in the treatment of several blood malignancies.

Research is ongoing to extend the use of immunotherapy to a wider range of blood illnesses, to provide long-lasting and minimally intrusive therapeutic alternatives. Furthermore, novel approaches to repairing genetic abnormalities causing inherited blood disorders are made possible by advances in genome editing technologies like CRISPR-Cas9. This offers hope for a solution to these conditions.

Furthermore, it is projected that the management of blood disorders will change significantly in the future due to the integration of telemedicine and digital health technologies. Teleconsultations, mobile health apps, and remote patient monitoring can improve patient participation in their care, make healthcare services more accessible, and provide real-time therapy response tracking. The movement towards decentralized healthcare models is consistent with the wider movement towards patient-centered care.

This approach emphasizes individualized treatment plans that take into account the patient's preferences and lifestyle in addition to the biological aspects of the disease.

Advances In Treatment

Treatment for blood disorders is changing dramatically due to new therapeutic approaches and a better knowledge of the underlying genetic and molecular causes. More focused and less toxic interventions are replacing and supplementing conventional treatments like radiation and chemotherapy, however, they are still necessary in some cases. A key component of the new therapeutic paradigm is targeted therapy, which is intended to selectively disrupt the molecular processes that underlie the onset and progression of blood diseases.

The treatment of certain blood malignancies has been transformed by immunotherapy, especially chimeric antigen receptor T-cell (CAR-T) therapy. With this method, a patient's T cells are genetically altered to express receptors that identify and combat cancer cells. A new standard in the treatment of cancer has been set by the approval of CAR-T therapy for several hematologic malignancies, thanks to its outstanding performance in clinical studies. Furthermore, monoclonal antibodies—which specifically target immune system components or cancer cells—remain effective in treating a variety of blood illnesses, providing more targeted and less harmful therapeutic options than conventional ones.

A vital therapeutic option for many blood illnesses, especially those brought on by genetic abnormalities or bone marrow malfunction, is hematopoietic stem cell transplantation (HSCT).

The success rates and hazards of transplantation have been greatly increased and decreased by advancements in procedures, such as better post-transplant care, reduced toxicity regimens, and improved donor matching. By expanding the pool of potential donors, alternative transplantation techniques like cord blood and haploidentical transplants solve one of the long-standing problems with hematopoietic stem cell therapy.

New Therapies

Emerging therapeutics have the potential to significantly change the management of blood disorders in addition to the known therapy approaches. Investigating gene treatments, which aim to repair or fix defective genes causing hereditary blood problems, is one such path. Leading this transformation is CRISPR-Cas9 technology, which allows for precise gene editing. Scientists are working hard to find a safe and efficient technique to use CRISPR-Cas9 to fix genetic abnormalities in hematopoietic stem cells.

This might lead to a one-time, cure for diseases like sickle cell anemia and thalassemia.

With an emphasis on utilizing the potential of antisense oligonucleotides (ASOs) and RNA interference (RNAi), the field of RNA-based therapeutics is likewise developing quickly.

By modifying gene expression at the RNA level, these strategies seek to offer a focused method of controlling the synthesis of proteins. Regarding blood disorders, RNA-based therapeutics are promising for diseases including some forms of leukemia and lymphoma that have aberrant or hyperactive gene expression. Positive outcomes from early clinical trials have opened the door for more research into these cutting-edge strategies.

Another class of novel treatments that target particular signaling pathways implicated in the onset and progression of blood diseases are small molecule inhibitors. Compared to conventional chemotherapy, these inhibitors provide a more tailored and focused approach by inhibiting important enzymes or proteins involved in the pathophysiology of the disease.

The continuous discovery of new targets and the creation of selective inhibitors can broaden the range of available treatments for different blood disorders, enhancing their effectiveness and tolerance.

Research Paths

The rapidly developing field of blood disorder research is directed in multiple important ways, all of which seek to close significant gaps in our knowledge of the underlying mechanisms of disease and enhance the effectiveness of current treatments. A crucial field of study is figuring out the complex genetic and epigenetic elements that lead to the emergence of blood diseases.

Next-generation sequencing technology and genome-wide association studies (GWAS) allow researchers to find new genetic markers linked to the development and susceptibility to disease, opening the door to more accurate risk assessment and individualized treatment plans.

Simultaneously, there is a growing focus on the investigation of the tumor microenvironment and the relationship between malignant cells and the surrounding tissues. Comprehending the intricate interactions of cancerous cells, immune cells, and extracellular matrix is imperative to create tailored treatments that impede the environment that promotes the advancement of the disease. Checkpoint inhibitors and cytokine therapy are two examples of immunomodulatory techniques that are being actively studied to harness the immune system and improve the effectiveness of current treatments.

Translating laboratory discoveries into clinically meaningful applications requires the creation of creative preclinical models and cutting-edge imaging technology. Organoids, three-dimensional culture systems, and patient-derived xenografts are being used more frequently to simulate the complexity of blood disorders in the laboratory, which makes it easier to find new therapeutic targets and assess how well drugs work. Furthermore, cutting-edge imaging techniques like magnetic resonance imaging (MRI) and positron emission tomography (PET) support early treatment response identification and non-invasive illness monitoring.

The optimization of efficiency and relevance of research endeavors in the field of clinical trials is being achieved through the integration of biomarker-driven methodologies and the trend toward adaptive trial designs.

Adaptive trials maximize the chance of discovering significant treatment effects by enabling real-time changes based on interim outcomes. Trials that are driven by biomarkers, which are defined by certain molecular or genetic traits, allow for more focused patient selection and raise the possibility of finding subgroups that benefit most from experimental treatments.

CONCLUSION

Thanks to developments in genomics, immunotherapy, targeted therapeutics, and a better understanding of disease biology, the area of blood disorder research is poised for unprecedented expansion and innovation. Personalized medicine, in which each patient's therapy is customized based on their unique genetic and molecular profile, is a promising development for the future. Immunotherapeutic interventions—in particular, CAR-T cell therapy—are changing the face of treatment for several blood malignancies, giving patients who had few alternatives in the past new hope.

New therapeutics are bringing us closer to curative interventions for inherited blood diseases and cancers. These include RNA-based strategies, small molecule inhibitors, and gene editing technologies like CRISPR-Cas9.

The amalgamation of telemedicine and digital health solutions denotes an additional paradigm change in favor of patient-centered care, with a focus on customized treatment regimens, accessibility, and remote monitoring.

A deeper comprehension of genetic and epigenetic variables, the tumor microenvironment, and the creation of sophisticated preclinical models will continue to propel advancement as research directions change.

therapeutic trials are becoming more targeted and efficient because of adaptive designs and biomarker-driven methodologies, which is hastening the conversion of scientific findings into valuable therapeutic applications.

All things considered, the future of blood disorder research is defined by the coming together of several disciplines, technological advancements, and a dedication to improving patient care.

By working together, researchers, doctors, and industry stakeholders can pave new paths in blood disorder diagnosis, treatment, and eventually prevention.

The path taken to get at these revolutionary results highlights the tenacity of scientific investigation and the steadfast quest to enhance the quality of life for those impacted by these intricate and difficult circumstances.